"*Plan for Tomorrow, Live for Today* is more than a book—it's a secular commandment. This guide to middle age exhorts the reader to change her life for the better. Think Daring Greatly meets Girl, Wash Your Face! Offering a surfeit of reliable sources, Wendy Campbell provides a clear recipe for any middle-aged woman to turn the next course of her life into a veritable feast."

—Aléna Guest, author of *Ravishing*

"What a shame I wasn't exposed to Wendy Campbell's sage advice decades ago when I was a mess in the romance department. If you're hoping to spruce up your partnership, delve into Wendy's lessons—you'll glean valuable information throughout."

—Alice Combs, author of *The Lady with Balls: A Single Mother's Triumphant Battle in a Man's World*

Acclaim for Wendy Campbell's Previous Book, *Personal Happiness*

"Being a woman in business has its own set of challenges. Being a woman in a male-dominated industry such as financial services adds even more to the list. Searching for that ever-elusive work/life balance makes this a perfect trifecta to address. Wendy Campbell's *Personal Happiness* hits it out of the park with her professional takeaways and personal stories. As someone who came through the same challenges with my own battle scars, I related to Wendy page by page. Opportunities don't always come gift-wrapped. Be open to those that are presented to you. Wendy's book is one opportunity to get your arms around."

—Judy Hoberman, President, Selling in a Skirt

Plan for Tomorrow, Live for Today

A Woman's Guide to Middle Age

Wendy Campbell

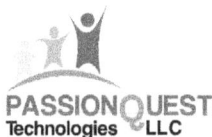

PASSIONQUEST
Technologies LLC

Plan for Tomorrow, Live for Today
A Woman's Guide to Middle Age
Copyright © 2020 Wendy Campbell

PassionQuest Technologies
5055 Business Center Drive
Suite 108, PMB 110
Fairfield, CA 94534
Phone: 707-688-2848
Fax: 707-402-6319
Email: info@earnprofitsfromyourpassion.com

PASSIONQUEST
Technologies LLC

Cover and book design by Cypress House
Front cover photograph courtesy of Jennifer LaRue Photography

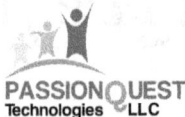

Publisher's Cataloging-In-Publication Data

Names: Campbell, Wendy (Wendy C.), 1975- author.
Title: Plan for tomorrow, live for today : a woman's guide to middle age / Wendy Campbell.
Description: First edition. | Fairfield, CA : PassionQuest Technologies LLC, [2020]
Identifiers: ISBN 9780991261154
Subjects: LCSH: Middle-aged women--Conduct of life. | Work-life balance. | Middle-aged women--Health and hygiene. | Self-actualization (Psychology) in women. | Interpersonal relations.
Classification: LCC HQ1059.4 .C36 2020 | DDC 305.244/2--dc23
Library of Congress Control Number: 2020944414

Printed in the USA
2 4 6 8 9 7 5 3 1
First edition

To all the women who enter middle age with grace and courage, free from the burden of others' judgments, and with the strength to be who you were meant to be.

God, grant me the serenity

    to accept the things I cannot change,

Courage to change the things I can,

And wisdom to know the difference.

—Serenity Prayer by Reinhold Niebuhr

Contents

Introduction

*D*espite the familiar saying, "In this world nothing can be said to be certain except death and taxes," change is also a sure thing. Along with changes in body, mind, and family and other relationships come huge changes and growth in heart and soul.

Acceptance is *"the act of taking or receiving something offered,"* not of just going through the motions. Take some time to evaluate how you got where you are. Assess what you can now change to never go back there again. Take some quiet time for yourself; become one with your prayers, your thoughts, your peace. Find something tangible and every time you touch it express gratitude for something that day, even if it's just for yourself. Expectations are premeditated disappointments; be realistic in your expectations and work within your limitations. Don't try to outrun them.

Accepting hardships as the pathway to peace is not simple or easy but it's possible if you commit to the journey.

Remind yourself that you're a work in progress—and so is everyone else. Believe true hope and inner peace are possible even when faced with hardships along the way. At midlife, as I step—often with ease and grace—into my fifth decade, I also stumble and nearly fall into it. In the not-so-distant past, I truly felt and believed I "had it all," success in every aspect of my life. Having it all implies an achievement of the final goal.

To believe there are no further goals, and having a rigid vision of success, often sets us up for a rude awakening because we cannot totally control our or others' behaviors.

Whether we embrace it or not, the very nature of change, growth, and enlightenment seems to come out of nowhere, often blindsiding us. This is the story of the past few years of my life. I now understand that my concept, my definition of success in my twenties and thirties, was minimal, structured, and "inside the box." Experience helped me understand that my own ideas often led me to be my own worst enemy.

Much of that experience has been difficult, heartbreaking, and far beyond my ability to control. Now, as I learn to embrace change, it's providing me the balance and harmony required to truly have it all, as much as I believe we can.

My intent with this book is to share what has empowered my journey—emotionally, spiritually, and intellectually—with readers who are also approaching or are in their forties. I invite you to join me in these pages on a path to self-discovery, change, and a new view of success.

Wendy Campbell
Fall 2020
Montrose, Colorado

Accentuate the Positive

*W*ho creates our boundaries? Is it us or are we allowing outside sources to do so? I used to be that girl—you know, the one who would not allow any other woman to penetrate my space physically or emotionally. That all changed as I approached middle age and my insecurities set in. My normal outgoing self would withdraw as I felt insecure. I would pull back and have the overwhelming feeling of a boundary being crossed. It took me a while to figure out that I get to make the rules and to decide if I am going to let "her" (or anyone else, for that matter) cross a boundary that they don't know exists. The bottom line became this: it's up to me to create a healthy boundary in order to not allow it to affect my attitude. This means I have to be reasonable in my thoughts and how I respond. Here's an example:

I walk into the room. I either own it or I let it own me. I either withdraw and let the catty woman in the middle of the room take over or I approach her with a sincere smile and engage. Easy to say, but hard to do—it's a constant effort to control our attitudes and not let others do so. By 40, we have reached an age where we have less and less time or energy to worry about other people and what they say or think.

It's easy to have a poor attitude. Our attitudes come from our thoughts, and when our thoughts are focused on the wrong things, we blame everyone and everything else, hold grudges, and don't know how to establish healthy boundaries. What if today we shift gears and work to turn every negative thought into a positive one; set and stand firm on our boundaries? How will our day change? Give it a shot!

A cup that's half full is quickly filled to overflowing by the choice to focus on the multitude of positive things in our lives. Throughout your day, stop frequently to take stock of all you have—of every little thing that makes your life truly wonderful.

I've heard it said, "If the mountain was smooth, you couldn't climb it." That statement has taught me a lot about trusting people, my friendships, good-byes, hellos, new beginnings, my family, anger, stress, and tested faith. Through it all, I've come to know this for sure: even in the happy and the painful, tear-filled, exhausting days, we need to remember we've done something right somewhere along the way.

As I sit at my desk this morning and look at the beautiful snowfall, I can't help but think of those who journeyed through a difficult previous year. The possibility of a new slate is welcomed by us all. For many, the year holds good memories and hope for the future. Others are relieved to see the year in their rearview mirror. Let's use the end of a year to foster an optimistic view: Reflection on the past year can bring us new ideas and goals for the year to come:

> Seek good health and happiness.
> Live one day at a time.
> Enjoy being in the present moment.
> Accept hardships as the pathway to peace.

I'm not perfect, and to acknowledge that is very important. I'm thankful that grace allows me to progress regardless and forgive myself for the times when I go about my day and "do life" without grace, even as I try to do better than I did the day before.

We all want to succeed in our work. Success in the workplace is determined by what we do there. Wherever "work" is for you today, make the most of it. Because success is measured in so many ways, only you can look back at the end of today and ask, "What did I accomplish?" Do your best to answer that and realize that your answer requires no justification by anyone but you.

Awareness Exercises

When I walk into a room, what's my attitude? Is it, "Here I am!" or do I step through the doorway and think, "Ah, there you are!"

Turning our attention outward takes practice and intention. Our culture offers us conflicting pressures. It exhorts women to be to be genuinely interested in others, yet we live in a consumer society that emphasizes self-indulgence and the acquisition of material things, a world that caters to our natural instinct to preserve and exalt ourselves. Let's switch things up. Instead of spending time looking for the perfect material acquisition or the perfect selfie, let's try to spend the bulk of our time focused on others. That will be more meaningful and more long-lasting. It's important to acknowledge our skills and talent, to bask in some praise, or post a photo on social media. Nothing wrong with posting an authentic, smiling photo. Your joy in the moment can be infectious and inspiring to others.

Next time you walk into a roomful of people you know, challenge yourself to have a meaningful conversation with at least three people. Listen deeply to each person. When you leave the room, take a moment to reflect on what you learned from (not necessarily about) each person.

Next time you plan to take a selfie, try thinking of it as a sharing of your joy or peacefulness rather than just a pretty picture or indulgence in a moment. And remember that your loving smile can boost the confidence of your friends and colleagues in person event more than it might online.

Discovering the Prime of Our Lives

*F*orty isn't exactly middle age nowadays. A forty-year-old today has a 50 percent chance of reaching age ninety-five, says economist Andrew Scott, coauthor of *The 100-Year Life.*

The number forty has a lot of mystical meanings: Jesus fasted for forty days and nights; Muhammad was forty when he saw the archangel Gabriel; the Israelites wandered the desert with Moses for forty years.

Age forty also feels important. An elderly English person said, "The forties are when you become who you are, and if you don't know who you are by then, you likely won't."

This is the age when we're supposed to be ladies and demonstrate that patience is a virtue. One forty-year-old *New York Times* reporter said, "When I try to act adorably naive now, people aren't charmed—they're baffled. Cluelessness no longer goes with my face. I'm expected to wait in the correct line at airports and show up on time for my appointments."

Let's be honest, once we reach our forties some tasks are harder. We get distracted easily, far more so than those younger women. We do not digest information as quickly, and our memories are not as sharp as they once were.

Our less-than-stellar processing power is balanced, though, by our maturity, insight, and experience. We have become so much better at recognizing the real meaning of a situation and knowing how to react to it. We're now able to resolve conflicts with dignity and grace and remain in control of our emotions. Our financial acumen has vastly improved, allowing us to make better decisions around money. As a rule, as we have approached forty, we have become more considerate than our younger selves and acknowledge the true blessing that is our happiness— we're less neurotic. Well, at least we try to be.

Let's look at this comparison as it applies to men in their prime. In describing men in this age group, Aristotle once said:

> ...they neither have that excess of confidence which amounts to rashness, nor too much timidity, but the right amount of each. They neither trust everybody nor distrust everybody, but judge people correctly.

Despite not being a man, I would have to say I feel I am there. My guess is that you are too! We have those qualities. We've lived, learned, and grown. We grasp the hidden costs of things. Our parents continue to give us unsolicited advice but no longer try to change us. We have finally reached a point where we are pretty comfortable in our own skins! Sure, we are always looking to change something aesthetically, but as a rule we are satisfied with who we have become.

Although we might still go for degrees, maybe find a new job, move to a new home, experience divorce, or the beginning of a new relationship, these events bring less awe now that we are in our forties. Our mentors and our moms and dads, who used to cheer our accomplishments enthusiastically, are becoming preoccupied with their own mortality. Sure, they still cheer us on and want the best for us, but we are not as important as we once thought.

We have this crazy notion that, if we have kids, we're supposed to marvel at their successes—and hey, that's not a bad thing! We will always hold that flag of pride high and discuss their successes and failures with our friends and coworkers; but life is changing, rapidly, and for the good.

We have done our jobs as moms, as those who "do it all"—and though we are still needed in other capacities, we have more to give to others by way of what we have learned. We can help others as we have been helped along the way.

When life feels out of balance, and you're looking for ways to cope, consider that within your church and your local community you likely have someone that you can sit with, cry with, scream with, or cuss with. This safe place to let your hair down is so very important. The person might not be a professional, but they can listen compassionately when necessary, and also tell you exactly what you don't want to hear (but need to). We all need someone who can give us these valuable reality checks. One can also look for online resources as a private way of seeking tools to deal with issues as they arise.

As we enter the world of middle age, we can still run companies, manage busy households, have classy benefits, and run marathons, yet there's something intangible about the age—plus an awareness of death—that wasn't present before. Some of our goals and possibilities feel narrowed. It's futile to pretend we're anything we aren't. That future life is no longer a dream. Our real lives are, undeniably, all about what's happening right now. That's right, my friends, we are able to start "living for today." We've arrived.

Finding Happiness at Middle Age

*W*hat does it mean to *"win?"*
Competition was important when we were young, and doing our best was usually at the top of our list of priorities.

However, it may be time to shift the mindset away from winning at all costs. You need not always try to be better than others. Instead, consider this: self-improvement should always be for the betterment of you and what you bring to the lives of others. Remember, you are good for no one unless you are good for you.

At this part of your life, you have made your place in the world—you are the real deal, an adult, and you have already won. Think about the stress of getting there, and what you did for that "win." You can let go of some or all of that pressure.

Try and think of yourself as a contributor instead of a winner. You are valuable and it's okay to think constructively versus focusing on how to beat or outshine other people. And you can now acknowledge a win with grace.

Our attitude can now be: "I will make my best contribution to those around me and allow others to do the same" versus "I will do better than everyone else." Make that contribution and stop worrying about other people. You'll feel a lot less stress and more happiness in the years ahead.

Stop right there! Stop comparing yourself to twenty-somethings who are worried about their place in the world and are busy obsessing over comparison with others.

Those days are over. Those young women lack experience. They're learning who they are, and they worry about measuring up. They have to look around and compare themselves to others, just like we used to.

They can't avoid it, but we can. Wouldn't it have been nice to tell our twenty-year-old selves, "Hey, just keep going, we know you already have what it takes and can face your own fears."

At midlife you've paid your dues and proven so much; it is important to look back and acknowledge that. We can appreciate our unique talents and appreciate others as well, without worrying about who is better. We have nothing to prove.

Focus on doing things you love, surround yourself with those who you love, and nurture those relationships.

It's time for self-expression, not looking for the approval of anyone. Many younger people will never admit it, but they long for both recognition and support. Remember this: if you're at midlife or beyond, there's no one better to approve of you than you. Twenty years later, we as adults look more outside ourselves to know we are all right. I wish I had the answer to why it takes so long but I don't—the reality is that it's past time.

It's time to become aware of your thoughts, your opinions, your feelings. Make a more mature expression of them, and watch the magic unfold.

When you finally come to realize that self-expression is more important than pleasing others, you will fully understand what a wonderful gift from the universe you have been given.

Some people will approve, some won't. Some people will love you, some will choose to ignore or dislike you. You need all of this to happen, because it's the real way to find people you can just be yourself with and not even think about approval. What a wonderful gift.

So, what is the gift? Simply being yourself in the company of people who appreciate you. This is the doorway to genuine relationships.

The alternative that is not ideal is to keep on moderating your thoughts and feelings and strategically putting yourself in just the right position so others will like you (or so you think). If they do actually like you, whom are they liking? Is it even the real you? They're only experiencing your façade, so it's impossible to really trust any approval you receive that way. Look at the amount of energy wasted on just going through those motions.

And, for what?

Being fulfilled in life means to be aware of and live by your personal values. This is especially important at midlife because that's when you're most capable of truly making use of your values.

What's most important to you in life? Your thoughtful answer to this question reveals your values. Read that question again and reflect on the ways in which you might answer it.

Create a list of your core values. Health, prosperity, freedom, love, security, being educated, peace of mind, friendship, clarity, balance...? Do any or all of these apply? What would you add, and in what order do they fall?

Our values should be the basis of any major decisions. Not sticking to your values in decision-making causes you to drift around in popular opinion and miss out on the joy that comes with doing what's right for you. It's not necessary to seek the approval of others—their opinion of you is none of your business (yes, that is exactly what you just read).

The secret to discovering your values is to forget what you think they should be and look for what they are, deep down. Take your time. You need to go really deep here.

One way to learn to do this work is with a therapist or someone in your life who you can learn from. Don't just focus on who this person might be, but also why you would want to work with them. When interviewing a potential therapist, ask them what their philosophy is – not just their therapeutic model or theories about human psychology. You're looking for a positive rapport with a professional who can help you assess your core values and acquire the self-knowledge that will serve you through thick and thin for years to come. This is a crucial emotional pivotal point! Some therapists will focus on your history and your family dynamics, others might focus on you as an individual.

Materialism May Be an Unconscious Self-Deprivation Scheme

We have spent years accumulating possessions which may have served as a way to increase our status and ego. We sought for proof we were worthy with external stuff.

Materialism is not a good strategy for happiness. In fact, people often obsessively seek things that don't bring lasting fulfillment at all. The car, home, clothes, jewels, gadgets, and toys excite us for a minute, and then that's it. Putting our stuff in a temporary gratification basket, we end up feeling empty, every single time.

"Stuff" is what it is, and can be enjoyed, right? When, however, you invest in stuff as your main means of happiness, it fails you big-time. No matter how hard you try to make it work, it will not be gratifying. You can stop. There is an awesome blog called "becoming minimalist" (https://www.becomingminimalist.com/). I've been following it on Facebook and found that I'm not just reading it but am putting the ideas and suggestions into action. Another inspiring and helpful internet resource is The Fly Lady (http://www.flylady.net). She can help you get organized and not feel overwhelmed in your own home. Both sites have great tips that you can subscribe to and get weekly or daily. They have helped me declutter my life.

My cousin gave me a copy of Donald Altman's book, *Clearing Emotional Clutter: Mindfulness Practices for Letting Go of What's Blocking Your Fulfillment and Transformation*; it's a must-read for clearing one's mind as well as one's space.

Acknowledge the Purpose and Presence of Authority

At midlife, do we stop resisting authority? The right answer is absolutely yes. If you have authority over your life, then you've agreed to the above. You are the Boss. Or, your boss has authority over you. Your job requires you to make some higher-level approvals and give direction. Okay, great, however by allowing those in authoritative roles just to do their job, you gain the following benefits:

- You get to relax and just do your function;
- You can focus on doing your best;
- You earn the trust of those with more power in any organization;
- The fact that you know your role reduces pressure; and
- Full responsibility for yourself is there.

It's time to let go of your struggle to prove you're better, smarter, or more capable than those with more authority than you. When you give up this chase, your talents and accomplishments will speak for themselves—and this is the key to rising in authority.

Settling In to Limitations

Limitations, however, are the crux of personal freedom. Let's talk about limitations. Not many people like to do so, but it's necessary.

> *The man with insight enough to admit his limitations comes nearest to perfection.*
>
> —Johann Wolfgang von Goethe

At midlife, you can free yourself from the illusion that

you are the all-powerful soul you once fantasized you were. This is much easier for women than it is for men, as you can imagine.

When you embrace limitations, you set yourself free.

There is always a balance between accepting limitations and growing. Only you know where that line is. And, to draw that line, you have to dig deep for the real answer, not the one you think people expect of you. So go ahead, draw that line.

Midlife might also be the time for you to develop clearer boundaries around what's acceptable to you. This can be done by understanding the incredible value of one simple word:

No.

- No, I can't go to the bar after work.
- No, I don't agree with you.
- No, you can't borrow my jewelry.
- No, I won't lend you money.
- No, I don't care for a movie.
- No, I won't clean up your mess.

No.

When you consider all the things on your list that you could agree with, commit to, or endorse, the list goes on and on. By knowing who you are and what's important, saying no maintains your integrity and your commitments. Not to mention the time it frees up.

Will people be offended? Not necessarily. That primarily depends on how maturely you deliver your message. The rest depends on the person receiving the message. "No" tends to sort out friends and supporters from the rest and simplifies your life immensely. Oh, if only I had known this sooner.

No discussion like this is complete without dealing with your view of your parents. In youth, you may have seen them as negligent or as oppressive and controlling.

Were they?

Now is a great time to begin to see them in a much easier way—as human beings. It's time to see the real value of our parents. They're merely people with their own strengths and weaknesses and struggles. Just like you.

Truly, at the end of the day, the answers you seek are found within you. We no longer look for outside assurance and status symbols. Every great thought leader in history has shown this principle to be true. Read the quotes below. Do you see the common thread?

The kingdom of heaven is within you.

—Jesus

Very little is needed to make a happy life; it is all within yourself, in your way of thinking.

—Marcus Aurelius

Since love grows within you, so beauty grows. For love is the beauty of the soul.

—Saint Augustine

Peace comes from within. Do not seek it without.

—Buddha

Education comes from within; you get it by struggle and effort and thought.

—Napoleon Hill

Each one has to find his peace from within. And peace to be real must be unaffected by outside circumstances.

—Mahatma Gandhi

Self-sabotage is a major issue. The same old problems and pain that are so familiar. In reality, it is the familiarity of all these issues that keeps us in a pattern of self-sabotage.

Open your eyes, look within. Are you satisfied with the life you're living?

—Bob Marley

Ladies, you have the tools, you are prepared, you are blessed.

The Importance of Healthy Practices

Taking Time for You Is Not Selfish, It's Necessary

*A*fter I hit forty, I spent some time figuring out what I was hiding behind. I looked at my vices and habits and decided what I wanted to change. My top ten health practices changed radically. Here's my new Top Ten.

- Stop taking my phone to bed; put it away when I am with others.

- Get adequate exercise and rest; listen to my body.

- Eat more protein and minimize sugars.

- Regulate my wine drinking.

- Use sunscreen.

- Keep positive company; minimize time with "Debbie Downers."

- Travel, Travel, Travel.

- Develop and practice a good skin-care regimen.

- Manage anger (with the help of a therapist).

- Spend time in the great outdoors.

You make sure you're getting good sleep, are being

sufficiently active, and are doing all you can to live a healthy lifestyle. At the same time, it's very important to make time to do the things you enjoy doing, fun and lazy things when you have some free moments. You can buy yourself a beautiful, small notebook and create a list right there of some things you would like to do but haven't taken the time for:

When can you start? Today is good. Obviously, you may not be able to do them all or get to it right away, but you have to make a point to start. What will it take to get you on your way?

Many people are finding the benefit in meditation, massage, prayer, or taking long walks. These activities:

- Boost your health;
- Increase immune function;
- Decrease pain;
- Decrease inflammation at the cellular level;
- Boost your happiness;
- Engender positive emotion;
- Decrease depression;
- Decrease anxiety;
- Decrease stress; and
- Improve your social life.

You may choose to do these things alone or in a social group, just make sure that if you do choose the group route you are among those who support your purpose and that you can likewise support their individual goals. Performing these actions in a group:

- Increases social connection and emotional intelligence;
- Makes you more compassionate;
- Makes you feel less lonely;
- Boosts your self-control;
- Improves your ability to regulate your emotions;
- Improves your ability to introspect;
- Changes your brain; it increases gray matter;
- Increases volume in areas related to emotion regulation, positive emotions, and self-control
- Increases cortical thickness in areas related to paying attention
- Improves your productivity;
- Improves your focus and attention;
- Improves your ability to multitask;
- Improves your memory;
- Improves your ability to be creative and think outside the box;
- Makes you wiser;

- Gives you a broader perspective: By observing your mind, you realize you don't have to be slave to it. You realize it throws tantrums, gets grumpy, jealous, happy, and sad—but it doesn't have to run you. This is simply mental hygiene: clear out the junk, tune your talents, learn to be at peace.

Sex Matters

*I*n a marriage or any committed relationship, sex can happen less often following the happy honeymoon phase. Life (as in "work"), concerns with new babies or grown children, health issues, erectile dysfunction, depression, boredom, a vibrator being more effective, letting oneself go, caring less about grooming or hygiene, relationship issues, medications that affect sex drive—all these can affect the amount of lovemaking time as well as its quality.

Honeymoons last anywhere from a few months to many, many years. If a "dead bedroom" sets in, and you both want to bring it back to life, you certainly can. Here are some ideas to think about and discuss with your loved one.

When you have something exciting, new, and adventurous in your life, the centers in your brain that release dopamine fire up powerfully. This is exactly what happens when you fall in love! Ballroom dancing and traveling to a fine vacation spot are great ways to form a bond and to increase the libido. Quality sex toys can also be fun, as are excellent, durable stimulators such as the Eroscillator.™

- Consider porn. There are different types, and some are quite classy, or funny, or entertaining. Read up on what's available and watch together.

- Study the Kama Sutra (an ancient guide to eroticism

and emotional fulfillment). Google is a good resource here.

- Stop the quickies—set aside time for leisurely encounters.

- Makeup sex seems nice, but heated discussions and conflicting opinions can work against your relationship. And never be wary of seeking counseling.

- Identify the issues together, and make sure you are both interested in solving the problems.

- Understand each other's position; be respectful even if when it's a struggle.

- Talk about potential solutions (options) do they make sense, are they obtainable?

- Decide on how you'll move forward

- Hold each other accountable for what each says they are willing to do. Revisit your conversation; just because tomorrow is better doesn't mean you've resolved an issue. Once you both agree that it is resolved, discuss how you might prevent things like that from happening again

- Work on fighting fairly and educate yourselves in healthy means of conflict resolution. Here is a good resource: therapistaid.com/worksheet/fair-fighting-rules.pdf

- Each of you writes a list of varieties of sexual play you'd like to do, then trade lists and decide together what you'll do that evening. This puts the focus on mutual desire.

- Spend some time mapping each other's bodies, touching various areas from head to toe, and writing down likes and dislikes. While you may think you know each other's wants and needs and areas of sensitivity, the mapping technique has enlightened many couples and drawn them closer through education.

- Nonsexual touching activity can be a good lead-in to sex. Massaging each other for an hour using quality scented oils can be fun and relaxing and a form of foreplay.

- Switch up your schedule—nighttime sex if you normally engage in the morning, or morning encounters if you're used to having sex at night. Enter into a few afternoon delights as well!

- If your partner is usually the initiator, don't be afraid to start the ball rolling yourself. It's always exciting and fun for the other person to be shown they're wanted and attractive.

- Trade roles. If one of you is more active in movement or always on top, change it up purposely; you may find that alone is quite a stimulating move.

- Dress up for sex now and then—a special new sexy nightie, some handsome new underwear or jammies—or you can go even further: use costumes and role-playing. All fun and helpful tools.

- Enjoy nonsexual adventures together, such as sports and movies, gatherings with friends, or travel. You'll see each other freshly in a new light when out with other people.

- Don't be concerned if your desire waxes and wanes; this is normal. Just stay in communication with your partner.

- Put sex on your agenda/calendar if it seems to not be happening enough. Scheduling and follow-through can make a difference.

- Arrive separately at a chic cocktail lounge, then sit at the bar pretending you've just met (as seen on TV's *Modern Family*), or do the same thing for breakfast at a diner counter. Carry through the pretending at home.

- Tease each other in a session of phone sex—even if you're just calling from a nearby room. Sexting can also be very arousing.

- Investigate local workshops in tantra (a slow form of sex believed to increase intimacy) or other sex-related topics.

- Book a weekend at a cabin or fancy hotel and pack all your alluring outfits and sex toys and books (try adamandeve.com or funfactory.com) so you can enjoy a sexcation holiday!

- Have a conversation to discuss each other's sexual fantasies.

Experts say talking about your masturbation habits can be very stimulating. You may have never discussed it, but most people masturbate. Talk about what you do to yourself that's most pleasing to you.

Being honest with your partner, and also kind, loving, and compassionate, can help overcome shyness.

Starting a Relationship in Midlife

*Y*ou've grown as a human being and as a partner for someone. You can avoid attracting partners who aren't worthy of your time. But, are you I ready to date? Are you ready to transition from single to attached again? Perhaps you have been in a relationship long- or short-term but are longing for something more. It's imperative to look at the dating options from the past as well as the present, and to stay mindful of "where do I begin to look when looking for common interest partners." Are you just looking for a sexual hook up or are you looking for actual companionship. Who knows, maybe that someone is all rolled into one. Knowing what *you* are looking for is more than half the battle. Be smart where safety is concerned, not only physical safety but emotional as well. Make sure someone of trust knows where you are headed and with whom. That may seem a little silly at this point in your life, but I assure you we are living in a world that we simply must be more pessimistic when it comes to "new people." Google dating sites and filter for what suits you, be honest in your description and proud of why you are there. There are so many things that have changed in the dating world in the last forty years, you can filter a lot while you drink a glass of wine in your fuzzy jammies long before you doll up for a night on the town with either Mr. Right or Mr. Right Now.

Regarding Game Playing

Who in the world has time for that nonsense? If you're mad, say so; if you're sad, say so; if you're grateful and appreciative, say so; if you want to pull your hair out and scream say so; but for heaven's sake don't play that passive-aggressive, poor-me game. Girlfriend, there is nothing more unattractive.

Coaches, programs, groups, and books can all be helpful in guiding you toward solid relationships. Time spent working on ourselves is a great idea before we enter the dating world. Do this, and you can bet on happier relationships. Getting back into the dating world needn't be daunting or distasteful. When developing a relationship, the most important thing you need for all concerned is to love and respect yourself.

When we're secure in ourselves, we attract secure people. Often the people we attract have issues like ours, so our own faults and foibles are likely to show up across the table from us on a date. If you often find yourself relating to people who need rescuing or mothering, take a step back and look at how you're presenting yourself.

Are you around these people because of your need to feel more secure and in charge? When we're secure, we attract secure people. Feeling insecure promotes anxiety and a longing for safety. Dating can trigger anxieties and challenge our confidence. We can stress over what to wear, what to say or not say, and how to say it. Practicing kindness and trying to be an interesting date are very good goals, but it's not good to be too invested in being what we think our date wants or in forsaking our authentic self. If you meet someone and wow, it seems like he could be the one, the ideal partner—please be careful, it could just be a passing physical attraction. Try to be patient and see how it goes for several dates. Dreams of "Love at first sight" can mislead us into wanting to be rescued from the unhappy parts of our past. We ourselves are the only ones who can help us get over what has been.

When you first start dating, you wonder where it'll go. What will happen after three months, six months, a year? Will this last? Some things you could consider I talk about in the next chapter. Some of these suggestions may seem pretty calm and boring, but remember: where we are in life, men are there too. If you want to make it last and have more than an occasional hook up, these activities can help you determine if you're likely to have a long, healthy, and happy relationship.

Can a Relationship be Depressing?

*H*ere are some things to think about if your relationship is not all that you'd hoped for.

Is Control an Issue?

Not having control over what happens in your relationship every day shows that your partner exerts more than their fair share of control. You should have an equal say in the basics, in your activities, choices, financial decisions, etc. If that is not the case, it needs to be discussed and changed.

It's Okay to Disagree or to Not Always be Pleased with Things

At times when your partner is angry, you can begin to feel isolated, which can be depressing. Not communicating with your partner will only make things worse and cause bad feelings. You have to be able to depend on your partner. If you can't, you will quickly find that it takes an emotional toll: it interferes with romance sex, creates difficulty with communication, is conducive to feelings of isolation, decreases motivation, fosters misunderstanding, and increases insecurity. It makes the relationship feel like a burden. None of those things are good.

Your relationship might feel like an albatross around your neck, making you feel immobilized and helpless. It takes great inner strength to recognize that the relationship is creating your depression, and then resolve to move on.

You Want to Fix Things, But Lack the Energy

You want a positive relationship with your partner, but the energy it takes to work on your problems seems out of your reach. Depression often creates a lack of physical energy that turns into mental paralysis that prevents your taking actions that might otherwise help you.

Contribution to the Relationship Has to be Two-Sided

Perhaps you do more around the house than your partner does, or he may provide more financially. There's sometimes an unequal distribution of work in a relationship, and it can make you feel sad or insignificant. If you're resentful of the imbalance but choose not to change it, you are part of the problem.

When Was the Last Time You and Your Partner Laughed…Together?

It is so important to fill your life with joy and positivity. Happiness is visible through the smiles and laughter loving couples share. If this positive emotional element is missing, depression might be occurring.

You Worry About Your Relationship's Future

If your relationship feels depressing, it can make you feel hopeless about the future. Being unable to see how your relationship could have a happy ending can make you worried, stressed, and sick, and the hopelessness can make you feel depressed as well.

Your Partner is a Poor Listener

A healthy romantic partnership requires good communication. Having no one to listen when you have a concern can lead to isolation and depression. Your partner should give you their full attention when you speak. If they don't, that lack of attentive listening can feel like a rejection, which leads to negative feelings and depression.

You Seek Someone to Talk to Outside Your Relationship

Confiding in someone else about how you feel about your relationship issues is a sign that you're not able to communicate with your partner, and such "emotional cheating" feeds the depression.

Learn to Just Be, with Nothing Pressing to Do

*Y*ou can relax and be comfortable just sitting around with each other, sometimes not even talking. Being able to just sit without conversation is a good sign.

If you argue and disagree, do it with consideration of each other and, in the end, maintain respect for each other's opinions. You can say you're sorry sincerely, but only if you are. At this point in life, it's okay to say, "I understand that you feel this way" not "I'm sorry you feel this way."

Don't use the silent treatment or name-calling—these habits are unhealthy. People in healthy long-term relationships find a way to make the other person feel heard and respected. Both men and women want a sound and quick resolution that uses constructive arguments without manipulation or hurtful tactics. Who has time for those games? We aren't teenagers!

Don't Expect Him to Have Your Back if You Don't Have His

In healthy, long-lasting relationships, the couple supports each other through good and bad, similar opinions, and differences of opinion. If you remain nonjudgmental with each other and put each other's needs high on your priorities, there's a strong chance you're a good match.

If you and your partner talk through things, you'll be able to support each other through life's challenges without judgment. Do you put each other's needs and happiness at the top of the "things most important" list? If so, then odds are the two of you are meant to be together forever. If you truly don't have his back or feel he doesn't have yours, have a discussion to discover where the relationship is really at. Clear communication about each other's expectations is crucial.

Share Friendships

Double dating can help build a stronger bond with your partner. Closeness with friends and spending time where personal stories are shared brings each couple closer. Hearing self-disclosure heightens feelings of passionate love, and the partners see each other more objectively and fully. We tend to be "ourselves" more so around our friends: what a great time to observe and be observed for who we really are when we are kicked-back in the company of friends.

Lots and Lots of Kisses

This isn't much of a shocker. Kissing is the distinguishing feature of all romantic relationships. As time goes on in a relationship, the importance of the kiss grows and becomes one of the most important things in maintaining a long-term relationship. The more you and partner like to kiss, the more satisfied you'll be with your relationship and the longer it'll last—go ahead, smooch away!

Laugh Out Loud

Laughter is the best medicine, just like the good-ol' *Reader's Digest* told us! It helps lessen depression, loneliness, grief, and despair. It makes us happy, lowers stress and blood pressure, boosts our immune system, and it fosters the closeness of two people or a group.

Laughing is one of the most important things a couple can do together. Do you laugh a lot? That's another sign you'll be laughing into old age together! If you're always serious or don't have a lot to giggle about, what good is that doing for either of you? Set aside some time to play a game together, read aloud to each other from an amusing collection of short stories, watch a rom-com together, go to a comedy club, or watch a (mutually) favorite sitcom.

Stay Honest

In committed, healthy relationships each has their partner's best interest in mind and at heart. Interactions are honest and direct. It's our goal to become closer and more connected. Games and manipulation are disconnecting—that, again, is teenage BS and should be avoided at all costs. Two classics in the pop-psychology genre that you might find illuminating are *Games People Play* and *You Are Not the Target*.

Nurture Respect

This is huge. Long-lasting love requires respecting each other's opinions, thoughts, work, talents, and time. Lack of respect and not being able to have honest, open talks can lead to resentment and ill feelings.

Be Grateful

Studies show that couples who express gratitude last much longer. Do you say things like "Thanks for picking up the groceries," "thanks for clearing off the table," "Baby, you just made my day!" or "I am so thankful that we met." If you do, you've chosen a path in life where love is your constant, your guide, and your future.

Are you a better person because of their support of your best self?

Self-improvements such as caring more about others, being on time, thinking before speaking, and being kind to those around you are all signs that you're in it for the long haul.

Mirror the Other's Vocabulary

You are not always going to agree with each other, but it is proven that if you and your significant other often use the same words, you have a higher likelihood of getting together and staying that way.

Snuggle Bugs

As if you needed another reason to cuddle. Spooning is a good sign! Studies show that couples who sleep less than an inch apart—and like to touch each other—are probably happier than those who sleep far apart. I personally prefer a queen bed to a king for that exact reason. The distance between partners in bed is thought of as demonstrating how a couple is doing while they're awake, so snuggle up for long-lasting love!

Equal Ground

It's hard to be in a healthy relationship when you have other people in your life trying to force their opinions on you or offering views and advice. Long-lasting couples do not allow people on the outside of the relationship to influence or control their relationship. Within your relationship you each can be in control of your own life without either of you dominating the partnership.

Trust is Everything

Without trust, there's no point in continuing a relationship. If you don't trust your partner, how could you create and maintain a long-lasting, happy relationship? There is a difference between "I trust you" and "I don't trust *her* around you." The only person you have to trust is your partner. There will be people who will push the envelope, cross that boundary, and make you question what's going on. But you don't have to trust them, you only have to trust your partner.

Distrust increases controlling behavior and leads to dissatisfaction. Full trust, on the other hand, allows both partners to be free to love each other honestly. And that, my friend, is bliss.

Health Always Matters!

G rowing older is a fact of life, but the way in which we age can largely be controlled by the day-to-day decisions we make. Bidding adieu to your thirties might mean that your body starts to tire more easily, and your schedule is likely full of everyone else's activities but your own, but that doesn't mean you should toss your needs out the window.

If you want to feel the way you did in your twenties or thirties (or at least try to), it's time to give your health a makeover. Here are some key actions you can take.

Match Your Workouts to Your Ability

You may have felt unstoppable in your prime, going for five-mile runs, miles of laps in the pool, high-altitude backpacking, and intense weight training, but as our bodies age, it's important to "go with the flow." Work with your local health club or a trainer to plan the best workouts and activities. Consider working with a dietician, too, to better understand your individual (and changing) metabolism, your current dietary needs and cautions. We will experience hormonal changes as we get older (such as more fat around our middles); this can change the way food is metabolized and the way our bodies use and produce energy. Take a good look at what you eat. Keeping an accurate and honest food journal for a week can provide a surprising amount of information and inspiration.

Balance Your Blood Sugar

I went to a nutritionist and had food testing done due to an autoimmune disease (rheumatoid arthritis/RA). It was by far one of the best decisions I ever made. It's called ALCAT testing; you can also get tested to eat correctly for your body type.

Though we might not call it a blood-sugar imbalance, we can feel when our blood sugar isn't well balanced. We might feel fatigued throughout the day, or wake up tired, or have an energy crash during our workday. Too often our solution is sugar or caffeine, but a better choice is protein. Something as simple as a little bit of cheese, chicken, yogurt, or even a Payday candy bar (which has as much protein as some of the expensive protein bars!) can solve the problem.

Diabetes is a disease that occurs when your blood glucose, also called blood sugar, is too high. Over time, having too much glucose in your blood can cause health problems, such as heart disease, nerve damage, eye problems, and kidney disease. You can take steps to prevent diabetes or manage it. An estimated 30.3 million people in the United States, or 9.4 percent of the population, have diabetes. About one in four people with diabetes don't know they have the disease. An estimated 84.1 million Americans aged 18 years or older have prediabetes. Changes in mood, energy, or sleep can signify that your blood sugar might be out of whack. A consistent and healthy diet can help us balance our blood sugar.

More information can be found at https://www.niddk.nih.gov/health-information/diabetes and https://medlineplus.gov/ency/article/002467.htm

Control Your Caffeine Intake

Too much caffeine can cause insomnia, irritability, and, when used as a quick fix for an energy dip rather than reaching for whole foods, you rob your body of a chance to fuel itself properly, which won't fix the underlying fatigue. As we age, some of us are getting up more often in the night to go to the bathroom. Studies have shown that women (and men) who drink more than two cups of coffee or soda per day were more likely to have bladder and urinary tract symptoms than those who did not; caffeinated diet soda appeared to affect women's symptoms at even lower consumption levels.

More information can be found at:
https://www.niddk.nih.gov/news/archive/2013/
feeling-what-you-drink

Don't Supplement Without Speaking to a Professional

It's easy to get pulled into the world of quick fixes and
"magic pills," but tread with caution when it comes to
supplementation. When you get your yearly physical, ask
your doctor to check your vitamin D level. You might find
that you need a supplement. Ask, too, about probiotics
and Omega-3 supplements.

For more information, see https://www.nutrition.gov/
topics/whats-food/phytonutrients

Sleep

When you were twenty, you might have gotten away with
getting only four- or five-hours' sleep, but those days are
long gone. You're likely being pulled in a million different
directions, but it's crucial to your health and sanity that
you get adequate sleep each night. Researchers are also
seeing a relationship between metabolism and sleep— "...
misaligning normal circadian rhythms with behaviors
such as sleep and eating—for example, by working the
night shift—increases vulnerability to diabetes, obesity,
and other metabolic problems. One likely reason for
these problems is the fact that the circadian clock has a
critical relationship with metabolic pathways important

to maintaining normal energy balance. For example, the synthesis of glucose (sugar) and fats and the release of glucose into the blood by the liver are governed by the circadian clock. Understanding how circadian rhythm and metabolism are linked therefore could help in the design of strategies to reduce vulnerability to metabolic diseases and is an area of intense investigation. (National Institute of Health)

Visit here for more information: https://www.niddk.nih.gov/news/archive/2013/time-sleep-metabolize

Cut Out Empty Calories Once and For All

One of the biggest changes we experience in our thirties and forties is how our bodies use and process calories. Jessica Crandall, a Denver-based RD, Certified Diabetes Educator, and National Spokesperson for the Academy of Nutrition and Dietetics, encourages us to eat breakfast in the first hour we're awake, and to eat something healthy every four to six hours.

She also says:

Focus on cutting out empty calories, because they add up quickly and don't leave you feeling full. Avoid wasting your nutrient needs on empty-calories items like chips, soft drinks, and latté syrups.

Make Your Diet More Heart Healthy

When you were younger the last thing you probably thought about was your heart health but being mindful of your ticker is very important as we get older. The earlier you make heart health a priority, the better because prevention is the most effective measure you can take. High-fiber foods and low-cholesterol foods, along with healthier fats and oils, can help make sure your heart stays healthy.

Kick Up Your Calcium Intake

Osteoporosis is a disease in which bones become fragile and more likely to break (fracture). It is the most common type of bone disease and increases the risk of breaking a bone. About one half of all women over the age of fifty will have a fracture of the hip, wrist, or vertebra (bones of the spine) during their lifetime. Spine fractures are the most common.

Your body needs the minerals calcium and phosphate to make and keep healthy bones.

- During your life, your body continues to both reabsorb old bone and create new bone.
- As long as your body has a good balance of new and old bone, your bones stay healthy and strong.

- Bone loss occurs when more old bone is reabsorbed than new bone is created.

Sometimes, bone loss occurs without any known cause. Other times, bone loss and thin bones run in families. In general, white, older women are the most likely to have bone loss.

Brittle, fragile bones can be caused by anything that makes your body destroy too much bone or keeps your body from making enough new bone. As you age, your body may reabsorb calcium and phosphate from your bones instead of keeping these minerals in your bones. This makes your bones weaker.

To maintain bone density, check with your doctor regarding the dosage if you're not able to maintain the optimum levels through diet alone.

For more information, see also
https://medlineplus.gov/ency/article/000360.htm

Vitamin B12

Older adults typically have a higher risk for vitamin B12 deficiency because our ability to absorb the vitamin decreases. We need 2.4 mcg every day. You can get this vitamin from meat, fish, poultry, milk, and fortified breakfast cereals. Some people over age fifty have trouble absorbing the vitamin B12 found naturally in foods. They may need to take vitamin B12 supplements and eat foods fortified with this vitamin. It's always a good idea to consult your health professional to make sure you're getting an adequate amount, and if not, they can suggest options for supplementation.

For more information, see also
https://www.nia.nih.gov/health/vitamins-and-minerals

Check Your Portion Size

Sometimes, changing our diet for the better is as simple as changing our table setting. Try eating a few meals each week from a single bowl, or from smaller plates. You'll likely be surprised at the number of calories you've saved! See also the *One Bowl Meals Cookbook* and *Buddha Bowls: 100 Nourishing One-Bowl Meals.*

Make It a Group Effort

You might feel like you're juggling everyone else's priorities but your own, but it's important to realize you don't have to go about your goals solo. Plan and cook a few meals each week with a friend or family member. Trading off the meal planning can save time and stress. You might consider a meal swap with friends for Sunday evenings to keep your taste buds intrigued. Meal delivery services such as HelloFresh, Home Chef, Blue Apron, Martha and Marley Spoon, can be helpful and inspiring, too, when getting together with friends.

Balance Your Needs with Demands on Your Time

Balancing work, family, exercise, and social life can be tricky. There are so many demands on our time these days. Take some time to reflect on how you'll organize each week so that you allow the time to take care of yourself, get adequate sleep, and make time for the things you enjoy doing.

Stay Connected with Friends

If you find yourself cutting short your runs or walks due to your busy schedule, frustration with lack of progress, or boredom, recruit a friend to join you in the activity. You'll often find the activity more inviting and entertaining and that you might take a longer walk or run. You can even call a friend to chat while you're walking if your schedules don't mesh. You might also find *Tiny Habits: The Small Changes That Change Everything*, by BJ Fogg, Ph.D., helpful.

Choose Community Over Complicated

It can be hard enough just to gather the whole family for a meal. If you don't have the time to make it from scratch, don't beat yourself up. Unless cooking complicated recipes is a relaxation for you, keep to the simple and rewarding recipes in your repertoire. Cutting back on the prep time will make achieving your health goals and that family togetherness that much easier. Take the time, spend the money on what works for you, then watch the magic of good health unfold. Find the protein that works for you; it's important that you eat the type you like and that it agrees with your body as it makes it so much easier to stay on track. Google "good proteins" for more information. There are many wonderful and inspiring cookbooks and cooking sites out there.

Here are a few favorites: Trim Healthy Mama at https://trimhealthymama.com.

These two sisters will teach you how to cook and eat for overall health, weight, hair, skin, and nails too. Their books and Pinterest ideas that follow Trim Healthy Mama are super user-friendly; with all the apps on our phones now there is no excuse for not having it all at our fingertips! I also recommend *Vegan World Fusion Cuisine, Thirty-Minute Vegan,* and other cookbooks by Mark Reinfeld (and Bo Rinaldi): https://veganfusionculinaryacademy.com/cookbooks

Talk to a Dietitian

What worked for you twenty years ago might not cut it anymore. When it comes to nutrition, don't forget to consult an expert to ensure that you're meeting the needs of your changing body. Let a dietician provide advice on options for both eating out and eating at home. If you haven't yet realized it, hitting the gym extra-hard won't undo the damage of that burger and fries the same way it did twenty years ago because your metabolism is slower. Get serious and start being more mindful and choosier with your food options. Fine-tuning your eating habits now will allow your body to function better in the long term.

Keep Moving, No Matter What

According to the National Institutes of Health, muscle strength and endurance are notably decreased with age. Muscle is at the end of the chain of events in movement, so virtually every step involved from oxygenating the blood to the delivery of oxygen to working muscle may contribute in some manner. The loss of strength, a hallmark feature of aging, may begin with inactivity. But one of the impressive features of skeletal muscle is its plasticity. This ability to adapt to its demands continues throughout our lives. The improvements come from central cardiovascular as well as peripheral muscle adaptations. Muscle is also fully capable of responding to resistance training. So, whether you're able to run, walk, swim, do yoga, or ride a bike—don't stop moving.

https://www.ncbi.nlm.nih.gov/pmc/articles/PMC3874224/

Start a Food Journal

If you've never logged what you eat, doing so might increase your weight-loss or fitness results tenfold. Food journaling is a good way to stay accountable to what you eat and how often you work out. By writing down your progress and reviewing it regularly, you can better assess your starting point and pick out any areas that may be holding you back.

Meditate

Going to the gym will strengthen your body, and meditating will work out your mind. Research published in *JAMA Internal Medicine* suggests that taking time to meditate daily can help reduce stress, anxiety, depression, and even pain. If you've never tried meditating, yoga can be a good practice to start with to help ease you into that type of mindful state.

Stop Avoiding the Doctor

It can be hugely beneficial to consult a trainer on matters of fitness, and to reach out to a dietitian to help create a healthy eating plan, but when it comes to basic health practices, you should see a doctor annually as a method of prevention.

Fill Up on Fiber

Less than 10% of most Western populations consume adequate levels of whole fruits and dietary fiber, with typical intake being about half of the recommended levels. Evidence of the beneficial health effects of consuming adequate levels of whole fruits has been steadily growing, especially regarding their bioactive-fiber prebiotic effects and role in improved weight control, wellness, and healthy aging. These potential health benefits include: protecting colonic gastrointestinal health (e.g., constipation, irritable bowel syndrome, inflammatory bowel diseases, and diverticular disease); promoting long-term weight management; reducing risk of cardiovascular disease, type 2 diabetes, and metabolic syndrome; defending against colorectal and lung cancers; improving odds of successful aging; reducing the severity of asthma and chronic obstructive pulmonary disease; enhancing psychological well-being and lowering the risk of depression; contributing to higher bone mineral density in children and adults; reducing risk of seborrheic dermatitis; and helping to attenuate autism spectrum disorder severity. Aim for over thirty grams of fiber per day. It's found in fruits such as raspberries, vegetables such as artichokes, whole grains such as farro and quinoa, and in beans, peas, and legumes.

https://www.ncbi.nlm.nih.gov/pmc/articles/PMC6315720/

Increase Your Potassium Intake

A low potassium level can make muscles feel weak, cramp, twitch, or even become paralyzed, and abnormal heart rhythms may develop. I'm not saying you need to double your banana consumption, but it's important that you consume adequate amounts of potassium. Potassium is found in a wide variety of plant and animal foods and in beverages. Many fruits and vegetables are excellent sources, as are some legumes (e.g., soybeans) and potatoes. Meats, poultry, fish, milk, yogurt, and nuts also contain potassium. Among starchy foods, whole-wheat flour and brown rice are much higher in potassium than their refined counterparts, white wheat flour and white rice. Milk, coffee, tea, other nonalcoholic beverages, and potatoes are the top sources of potassium in the diets of U.S. adults It is estimated that the body absorbs about 85%–90% of dietary potassium.
https://ods.od.nih.gov/factsheets/
Potassium-HealthProfessional/

Sleep

Be gentler and kinder to yourself—you deserve it! At age twenty, four or five hours of sleep may have worked for you, but alas, not anymore. You're super-busy now, so it's crucial to your physical and mental health to schedule enough restful sleep each night. Seven or eight hours is the norm to guide you.

Modify Your Workouts

No need to ditch your past exercise routines—you can adapt them to your forty's life. Perhaps shorter runs and fewer sets—see how it goes and watch the scale. Lower-impact options such as cycling or the use of lighter weights and more repetitions. Keep in mind that strength or resistance training is more effective than cardiovascular activity in the preservation of precious muscle mass. For knees and hips that have been overused, water jogging and running, deep or shallow, is especially effective.

There's Nothing as Certain As Change

*C*hange happens throughout our lives, but some real knock-your-socks-off changes occur as we enter and move through our fourth decade.

One is that the kids are suddenly all grown up. They're young adults, and are off at school, or if that's completed, maybe they're starting families of their own. They don't need a mom as much anymore. Best case scenario: a closeness—genuine friendship—remains always.

If motherhood has been the central part of our lives, as in having been stay-at-home moms, the adjustment to an empty nest can be extra-difficult. When the kids have gone, outside activity such as volunteer work or a paying job can help us transition. Staying at home as we did in the child-rearing years is not at all therapeutic. It's time to take charge and find new sources of fulfillment.

Men aren't often good at helping us through this sense of loss. We can help ourselves and our mates adjust and delight in our new freedom by suggesting fun dates and other activities that add spice to a marriage or partnership: Take long walks, try a dance class, watch movies at home or in a theater—with coffee-shop discussion after. Go to concerts, enroll in a painting class, or take up a new sport—pickleball is the rage right now. Learn a new card game together and join a group that plays it. Find a home project to get involved in—redecorating, perhaps, or downsize to a smaller home, cottage, or condo.

For you, spend more time with girlfriends; many will be in the same boat as you, but focus the conversations on today and tomorrow, not on commiserating about the children being gone.

What both mom and dad might look forward to from the children is texts, phone calls, holidays, dinner visits back and forth, and the future possibility of sons and daughters-in-law and enjoying their grandchildren.

Meanwhile, if the life changes seem too tough to handle, it's wise to seek professional help—therapy can make a huge difference in how soon you feel great again.

During the forties decade, there are other changes that impact life as much as the children leaving. Remember: You're not old, you still feel invincible—in your prime—but subtle new issues arise. According to widespread health sources:

- Metabolism: Slows 2% per decade.
- Muscle: 6 to 7 pounds less of it than ten years ago.
- Bone: Since your mid-thirties, drops by 1 percent per year.
- Libido: Elevated stress levels and hormonal changes can lower it.

- Stress: Caused by concerns about kids, aging parents, health, career, and finances.

- Depression: More likely now.

The following habits can keep you healthier and thus happier though your forties and beyond.

Always Have Breakfast

It's essential to keeping metabolism up and weight down. Reason: A solid meal at the start of the day works with your metabolism. It's your fuel and prevents low blood-sugar cravings. A couple of good meal examples:

Overnight Oatmeal. At night, mix a half cup old fashioned oatmeal and a half cup of fat free or almond milk in a large mug with 1 tablespoon maple syrup. Refrigerate. In a bowl put 1 cup frozen mixed berries or cherries to defrost all night in the fridge next to the mug of oatmeal. In morning, cut up half a banana and add it along with the berries to the oatmeal mixture, with more milk if desired.

Chocolate Smoothie. Mix ½ cup milk, 1 tablespoon unsweetened cocoa, 1 cup frozen blueberries, 1 tablespoon ground flax, 1 cup fresh spinach, and half a frozen banana in a high-speed blender. Blend till smooth and pour into a tall glass. Drink on the go if you wish.

Boost Your Metabolism

Strength-training at a gym or at home can strengthen bones, improve balance, and prevent injuries—important for now and moving forward. Exercise at least thirty minutes most days of the week. Consult experts in the field on what program is best for you.

Boost Calcium and Vitamin D

Both are essential for strong bones. For women in their forties, the National Osteoporosis Foundation advises 1,000 mg of calcium daily. They also recommend 400 to 800 IU of vitamin D every day, from foods such as milk or salmon. Check the foundation or a registered dietitian or nutritionist for the latest figures.

Keep Stress Levels in Check

Stress is conducive to faster aging. The unhealthy changes brought about by stress include heart rate issues, increased blood pressure, and reduced energy and strength. A healthy, calm heart beats faster when you inhale, slower when you exhale, but stress puts a damper on this variable heart rate, causing unhealthy changes over your whole body. These include increased blood pressure, less brain capacity, reduced sex drive, and faster cell and molecular death. Sounds awful, right?

So, here's a simple task you can do every day to help.

A De-stressor Tool: Count to 4 as you inhale through your nose, then exhale for an 8 count. Do this twice a day as a regimen, and anytime you feel stressed. Doctors affirm that the vagus nerve, which runs from brain to pelvis, serves to relax the heart, muscles, airways, gastrointestinal tract, and blood vessels. Sexual activity with the one you love (even if it's you alone!) is a tried and true way to relieve stress.

Protein: A Closer Look

Dietary proteins are not all the same. They are made up of different combinations of amino acids and are characterized according to how many of the essential amino acids they provide.

- Complete proteins contain all of the essential amino acids in adequate amounts. Animal foods (such as dairy products, eggs, meats, poultry, and seafood,) and soy are complete protein sources.

- Incomplete proteins are missing, or do not have enough of, one or more of the essential amino acids, making the protein imbalanced. Most plant foods (such as beans and peas, grains, nuts and seeds, and vegetables) are incomplete protein sources.

- Complementary proteins are two or more incomplete protein sources that, when eaten in combination (at the same meal or during the same day), compensate for each other's lack of amino acids. For example, grains are low in the amino acid lysine, while beans and nuts (legumes) are low in the amino acid methionine. When grains and legumes are eaten together (such as rice and beans or peanut butter on whole wheat bread), they form a complete protein.

You can get a mood-lifting brain boost by eating complete proteins twice a day. This helps relieve such symptoms of depression as slow thinking and dulled memory. Current thought is that a sedentary adult woman needs roughly .4 grams of protein multiplied by her weight in pounds, and active women need .6 grams of protein for every pound of bodyweight.

According to the CDC (Centers for Disease Control and Prevention) the average American woman aged 40–59 now weighs 176 pounds. Thus an average sedentary woman would need about 70 grams of protein daily, while her active counterpart would need 105. By contrast, a sedentary 130-pound woman needs 52 grams of protein, and her active counterpart needs 78 grams (28 grams = 1 ounce).

Go Out with Your Girlfriends

According to Edward Schneider, M.D., professor of gerontology and medicine at the University of Southern California's Andrus Gerontology Center: Relaxing with friends reduces stress, boosts self-esteem, and even makes you more loving toward your partner when you get home. Women are terrific at connecting socially but often let it fall by the wayside in their 40s because of career and family demands. Women with extensive social networks through family, work, volunteer organizations, religious groups, or hobbies have lower blood pressure, less diabetes, reduced risk of heart disease, and half as many strokes as women who are less well connected.

Get Essential Checkups

We should not neglect these:

- Eye exam: every 2–4 years
- Blood pressure: every 2 years
- Pap test and pelvic exam: every 1–3 years
- Thyroid: every 5 years
- Mole check: every year
- Mammogram: every 1–2 years
- Blood glucose: every 3 years starting at age 45

Source: Office of Women's Health, US Department of Health

What You Say and What You Don't Say Can Make a Difference

*F*or now, I want to help you with the "not say." If you've ever felt miserably uncomfortable with a man when it got quiet, I know how you feel. There isn't a woman on the planet who doesn't squirm and feel weird when things suddenly go silent—but it needn't be awful. In fact, you can use the silence to your advantage with a man, if you know how, because sometimes—often, in fact—nothing is the right thing to say.

Sometimes, just letting there be *air* between you, and breathing, and being quiet is the way to go. Sometimes, you want him to *feel* you rather than *hear* you.

Most important, you want to be able to hear those weighty voices inside your head that are yelling; trying their hardest to make you do something that could damage whatever wonderful thing might be happening in a moment of blissful silence.

We Must Love Ourselves Before We Can Be Loved by Someone Else

*F*or a happy life and great relationships, we have to love and accept ourselves fully.

Our partners might say, "I love you so much" and we won't completely believe them. We'll be a little paranoid, and think we're not loved.

If they didn't call when they said they would, we think it's because they don't love us.

Did they suggest sex, or cuddle, or hold our hand as we walked down the street? If not, we think they're losing interest.

We're reluctant to tell them our secret feelings or fears, because that would push them away.

We feel like we're not "good enough" to go out with our dream date, or we settle for someone who's "fine" but doesn't make our heart leap with joy.

We mistrust our partners—think they're lying and cheating on us.

We carry around the feeling that we're never good enough to have the love other people experience. We doubt ourselves, our partners, love—we doubt everything.

We let challenges deflate us, we have a low opinion of ourselves. We never ask for a raise; we stay in dead-end jobs.

We lose weight only to regain it and then some. We give up on our health, saying it's too much effort.

Quick fixes are our MO to feel better: a new hairdo, a one-night stand, a bottle of bourbon, a hot-fudge sundae, but none of that works—we feel lonelier, emptier, sadder, and we'll stay that way till we accept and love ourselves and stop looking for others to give us the love and caring we yearn for.

Because if we don't think we are worthy, why should anyone else?

Know that loving yourself changes your life more than anything else you can do.

Until we do it, we don't realize how powerful it is.

We do whatever we can to avoid looking inward, because it's intimidating; it means affirming our sadness, remembering past hurts, and facing our fears.

We reject self-love instead of embracing it as the uplifting force it can be.

We use our credit cards, our five-star meals, our mediocre relationships, and wrap ourselves in their protective cocoon in place of acknowledging how we feel inside.

Loving yourself means you reveal who you really are. You share your feelings—even the embarrassing ones—and own up to the truth of your life and your mistakes.

You needn't prove anything to anyone, because you know the only opinion that matters about your self-worth is your own.

You've learned to refuse to accept bad treatment, or social pressure, or feeling compelled to do things you don't want to do just because you're "supposed to."

You can now fully accept and enjoy being loved by someone else. You don't doubt their feelings. You never worry if the love will end or if you aren't good enough. Not anymore!

You aren't afraid of getting hurt. You don't push love away, or run away, or think up reasons why your relationship will let you down.

You are at peace with you and can channel your energy into creating what you want instead of protecting what you don't want to lose.

You feel excited, light, and free!

Silence Isn't Always a Treatment

Silence can embrace a loving moment or be a destructive and manipulative act. Humans communicate with eye contact and body language, not just words. Scientific studies have shown that most of human communication is nonverbal. Silence doesn't mean someone is angry, disinterested, or upset. Sometimes we're distracted by something that happened earlier in the day or we're planning for an upcoming event. Perhaps we have an upset stomach, or a toothache, or we're just plain tired. Sometimes we just need a moment alone. When your partner is silent, rather than imagining all the negative possibilities a simple request—"Tell me what you're thinking of right now"—can pave the way to deeper communication. We can indeed stay emotionally connected even during silent moments.

God gave us one mouth and two ears for a reason. At the first sign of silence, our hearts start thumping and we go into panic mode; we assume the worst and we get fearful. But don't make the mistake of trying to fix something that's likely not broken. Take a deep breath and look at him with loving eyes.

More of us need to realize that *silence can be bliss!* It can strengthen your relationship when you understand that you can just sit and "be." It's not necessary, or wise, to speak just because the silence makes you uncomfortable.

Practice breathing—in and out, in and out. Look out the window, or at other folks, or at the TV if it's on. Important point: refrain from resorting to fiddling around with your phone!

You could pull a snack from your purse, offer him some, and munch very slowly. Try putting your hand warmly on his arm, or his knee if you're close. Smile just as happily as you feel in that moment. Consider taking a walk together and not speaking until you're bound homeward or back to the car. Don't start reading a magazine, don't pick up your phone. Instead, notice what's going on in the room around you. Look calmly out the window or continue quietly watching the movie. You might fix yourself something simple to eat and snack on it slowly.

Now that you're relaxed, the right words can just pour out naturally. Talk to him—and more important, listen. Be accepting of another silence if there is one. It won't be awkward, and it won't last.

If you notice that you're physically reacting to his silence in a negative way, you can work your way out by grounding yourself. If you're standing, balance your weight as evenly as you can between your feet. If you're sitting, move toward the front of your chair and lean forward a bit. Inhale slowly, then exhale even more slowly. You'll likely feel calmer in just a moment (there are scientific reasons for this – it's not just a theory). If you still feel anxious, try to focus on your belly, just below your navel and put your hand there. Take another deep slow breath and let your belly expand into your hand. Next, where are your shoulders? If they're hunched up around your shoulders, let them drop. They're not earrings! With your next exhalation imagine your love traveling across the room to him as you help create and nurture a safe place for both of you to be vulnerable and open.

When Your Kids Grow Up

*T*ime has a way of playing tricks on parents. When we're in the thick of motherhood, we feel like our kids will be little forever. We're always running on EMPTY, going a mile a minute, taking care of our children and tending to the house. We're just trying to survive—doing our best to make it through another day. Our kids are always together, fighting in the hallways, giggling on the couch, making a mess through dinner, running around, and needing our attention. We grow so used to having them there that it's hard to imagine a day when they aren't.

Then one day you wake up and your kids are gone. They may be off to college or have joined the military or got their first apartment. Their rooms sit empty, their beds always made. No toys on the floor, no giggles echoing through the halls, no fights to break up. Their chairs are bare at dinnertime. The laundry baskets are empty, and the kitchen is clean.

Their absence is everywhere; the silence is deafening. The heartache is real, and anyone who says it's not is full of crap. You wonder how the heck it happened, because eighteen years is a long time, right? How could it be over already? It hurts. You spend your whole life preparing your children to leave home—as they should—but no one prepared you for how you'd feel when that day came. You never thought it would come so quickly. You thought you'd have more time, another day, one more chance, but time sneaks up on you when you're not looking.

Though all this is sadness is a reality, the time has come to celebrate your children's newfound direction alongside them. It's time to find your new normal, to create a deep appreciation for this new adult family time with a grateful heart. Smile at their successes, cry privately about their struggles—it's all part of the deal. They still need us, but in a whole new capacity. Find your lane and *stay in it.* Guide them through conversation, don't dictate and talk at them. It's important that they come back to you with the next challenge to work through and the next success to celebrate. It makes your new time together all the sweeter.

Even after divorce and starting a new blended family, I smiled at the sight of our four grown children, laughing, smiling, getting to know one another as they kicked off their shoes and dropped their bags in a spare room to stay the night with us. When they open the fridge and make themselves at home. When they give me a big hug. Our children are what makes a house a home—what fills it with warmth and laughter and love. I know this is what we will one day refer to as the "good old days," the days we never forget and always look forward to, these days when we're all together, home, under the same roof. Over time, those occasions become fewer, then become different, but they're always good, and we should always welcome the "kids" with the acknowledgment of where they've been, where they are now, and where they will be. This comes with growth of their own families and watching them create their new normal. Nurture it, support it, and enjoy the moments that are truly priceless.

How to Have Something Special and Everlasting

*C*onsider this: It truly is the little things that make a big difference.

Greet him warmly: when he comes home; when he enters the room; when he's nearby.

Offer a kind word. There's a lot to be said in a kind voice.

Thank him for the life you get to share together and for all he does to make it good.

Speak the truth. In love. Always.

Look at the bright side. Focus on all that's good and right. Sometimes we need to remind him of this too.

Let irritating habits bounce off you. Shrug off small annoyances

Snuggle together whenever you get the chance. Mostly because it's fun.

Serve cheerfully, even if it's fallen out of fashion. Some of Grandma's habits are hard to break: don't hesitate to fix him a drink and encourage him to kick back and tell you about his day.

Pray for him. Whomever or whatever you pray to, pray for his health and overall well-being. It really does make a difference.

Listen carefully. About his day, his worries, and his dreams. Support them. Ask him to tell you something random.

Apologize humbly. Be quick to say you're sorry and ask forgiveness when you're wrong (yes, occasionally we are).

Kiss on the lips. And then linger, like you mean it—nothing wrong with time spent that way.

Laugh at his jokes, even if you've heard them before, even if they're not funny.

Give a soft answer to all the questions he asks. Always listen and respond, but don't just listen to respond—there's a difference.

Step away together occasionally, far from the world and its pressures, just the two of you.

Smile at him. Smile with all your heart. Light up whenever you see his beloved face. This should come naturally. Don't force it.

Put his past and your past completely behind you, never to be brought up again. Easy to say, doing it is key.

Spend time together every chance you get but find opportunities to give him space and encourage him to spend time with his friends or alone. Don't forget to do the same for yourself—it's important to miss each other.

Build him up rather than tear him down. You'll never be sorry for doing so.

If you've decided you're going to love each other for the rest of your lives, then congratulations are in order!

Now go make every day count by living and loving as if tomorrow might not come.

Marriage Versus Commitment

*C*ommitment is vowing that you're in this relationship for the long haul. It's promising that your relationship is a priority, and you'll do what it takes to nurture it.

Emotionally Naked

It's more important to be someone's everything than it is to hold a traditional title of "Marriage."

Let's talk candidly about marriage versus commitment.

Don't leave this world without experiencing the joys of committed relationship—it's the most glorious garden you'll ever discover.

Want to be truly happy in a relationship? This is far more important than saying "I do."

How do you feel when you hear the statement "Married people are happier?"

If you're married and struggling with your spouse, you might feel like that whole idea is a cruel joke. *How come I'm not so happy?*

If you're in a relationship but not married, you might feel offended, even angry. *Who says a piece of paper really means that much?*

If you're single, you might feel marginalized, depressed, even defective. The love you long for hasn't yet appeared, and you despair that it ever will. *So, are you saying I'm unhappy just because I'm not married?*

Well, here's the good news: all those studies and conventional wisdom are getting something seriously *wrong*.

Commitment fears show up even in the most "committed" relationships; your underlying commitment fears may surface in you or your mate as control, bickering, the need for space, and even bedroom troubles.

Yes, people in happy marriages are generally happy, but it's not the fact that they're married that makes them happy.

Being "married" is a status—a status that means nothing if the traditional and religious aspects mean nothing to you.

Something underneath that relationship status is the actual engine behind happy couples. Ever wonder what it might be? I look at it like this: A relationship is like a garden.

Think of a harmonious relationship as a carefully tended garden. This garden has many benefits: beauty, peace, tranquility, safety. This is where true intimacy can grow. Only when you're in the garden do you get to enjoy and experience all of it.

The catch, however, is that the garden gate is locked.

The key to that gate is commitment. Only commitment unlocks the gate and lets you into the garden. Commitment defined: "You and I agree to maintain this garden so that it is always in bloom; if we don't care for the garden, it will wither and die." This beautiful garden of intimacy isn't opened just because you're married. It's opened because you're willing to do what it takes to keep it alive and growing; willing to tend it and nourish the soil and seeds; to savor its beauty, celebrate its gifts, and spend time in it regularly.

You'll put it back together after a damaging storm—with the power of recommitting to your partner. You see, commitment gets you in the game (and in the garden!), but recommitment keeps you in it. In short, you commit to the garden's well-being, and as a result you get to enjoy all of its many blessings and the happiness it bestows.

"Doing what it takes" also means closing all the backdoors and side doors to the garden: If you threaten (or even entertain) separation when conflict occurs, you haven't fully committed.

If you secretly fantasize about being with someone else, you're not fully committed.

If you think, "Let's take this day by day and see if it works out," you're not fully committed.

If you've given yourself any kind of out, you're not fully committed.

If you have one foot out the door, then you're not

harnessing all your resources to create lasting, genuine love. It's that simple: if you're all in, then you get to enjoy all the benefits of the relationship—*because your commitment is what makes those benefits possible.*

Your mutual commitment is what creates the safety and trust you both need to fully love each other.

You don't spend time worrying that what you say or do might scare this person off.

You don't hold back the best of you to protect yourself from getting hurt. You're not afraid to share even your most difficult thoughts and feelings.

You can rest in the knowledge that your relationship is a safe haven where both mistakes and growth are possible.

Without commitment, you don't get to enjoy all the garden's benefits—you're just an onlooker, standing outside the gate looking in. Commitment is the catalyst to trust and intimacy. It helps us prevent our fears and past hurts from sabotaging our happiness.

We all enter into relationships with fears and barriers to love. You might be afraid that if you get too close to someone they will hurt you; or if someone truly gets to know you, they won't like what they find; or that a person will change—like all the other people you've dated have—and leave you disappointed and alone again. Commitment unlocks the barriers to love you might have, because until you make a real commitment to someone, you can't be fully vulnerable. If either of you has one foot out the door, you can't fully trust that you and your relationship are safe, but once you've committed to making this relationship work, you're safe to become emotionally naked with each other; to share these fears and past hurts and secret desires. You're safe to express scary emotions and truly welcome someone else into your life; to consider the needs of the relationship as equal to your own. When you can count that your partner is committed to deepening the connection you share and willing to accept the messy parts, you can begin to heal the inner parts of you that feel unworthy or unlovable. You're no longer reacting to the fear of being abandoned, and instead put your energy into loving each other... no matter what.

Marriage Doesn't Equal Commitment

You can be married and yet be uncommitted—I can speak to this firsthand, and I'm sure you've seen it too. Affairs, workaholism, and unilateral decision-making are all examples of keeping one foot outside the garden gate. Refusing to accept equal responsibility for relationship issues is also a sign of noncommitment. That's why marriage in itself isn't what can make you happier, and it isn't what makes a relationship. Commitment is the door opener to relationship happiness—married or not. What matters is whether you've committed and closed all the exit doors.

I'm not saying marriage isn't wonderful—it *can* be, but I want you to understand that it's not relationship status that fuels the happiness; it's commitment to the relationship. Marriage can give your commitment power, but it doesn't power your commitment.

Commitment is an art, and it's one we all *must* learn. Many of us grew up without appropriate role models for what true commitment looks and feels like, so we mistake marriage for commitment; or we lack the tools to make our marriage work once we get there. Some of us grew up with ideal role models and still made the choice to be "uncommitted." If you want your relationship to flourish, one of the most important steps you can take is to learn how to truly commit—it's the only way you'll fully experience the love and joy a relationship can bring.

Making a meaningful commitment is more than just saying, "I commit." There's a way to bring it deep into your body and align it with what you want in life—today and tomorrow. Moreover, there are specific tools and actions you need to take to make that commitment last, so what you want deep in your heart can become a lasting reality. If you're married, in a relationship, single, or anywhere in between, commitment is the life force that will power all your relationship happiness. It's the first step you need to take if you want love to last. Skip it, and your relationships will wither and die—or worse, continue in a state of inner longing. In order to keep commitment strong, you'll need to get into the habit of expressing your thoughts and feelings—even the most difficult ones.

Selected Resources

- http://www.flylady.net
- https://medlineplus.gov/ency/article/000360.htm
- https://medlineplus.gov/ency/article/002467.htm
- https://ods.od.nih.gov/factsheets/
  Potassium-HealthProfessional/
- https://psychcentral.com/blog/
  silence-the-secret-communication-tool/
- https://www.accessdata.fda.gov/scripts/Interactive-
  NutritionFactsLabel/protein.html
- https://www.becomingminimalist.com/
- https://www.havetherelationshipyouwant.com/m/
  email/nl/silence-creates-love.html
- https://www.helpguide.org/articles/relation-
  ships-communication/nonverbal-communication.htm
- https://www.ncbi.nlm.nih.gov/pmc/articles/
  PMC3874224/
- https://www.ncbi.nlm.nih.gov/pmc/articles/
  PMC6315720/
- https://www.nia.nih.gov/health/
  vitamins-and-minerals
- https://www.niddk.nih.gov/health-information/
  diabetes

- https://www.niddk.nih.gov/news/archive/2013/feeling-what-you-drink
- https://www.nutrition.gov/topics/whats-food/phytonutrients
- https://www.theverge.com/2017/3/30/15109762/deep-breath-study-breathing-affects-brain-neurons-emotional-state
- therapistaid.com/worksheet/fair-fighting-rules.pdf

About the Author

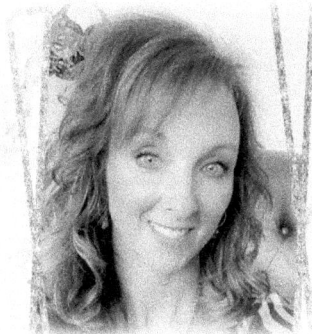

*W*endy Campbell, a small-town girl with big-city dreams, had a twenty-four-year marriage and is the mother of two. A successful insurance and financial entrepreneur since high school, as well as a speaker and author, she lived in a small ranching area and raised her children amidst close family while she served neighboring communities in her business and as a volunteer. Wendy has a blended family of four, and recently relocated to Montrose, Colorado.

While facing tough challenges as midlife approached, Wendy learned invaluable lessons. She tapped into her business experience as she continued her entrepreneurial journey, and found her passion in the Wellness industry. She has recently launched the Montrose Day Spa & Wellness Center. Among the uplifting experiences of recent years was the thrill of welcoming her first grandchild, lovingly nicknamed Peanut. The icing on her midlife cake: Wendy is blessed to have found her soulmate.